4 first place
health

my food plan

Published by Gospel Light
Ventura, California, U.S.A.
www.gospellight.com
Printed in the U.S.A.

Caution: The information contained in this book is intended to be solely for informational and educational purposes. It is assumed that the First Place 4 Health participant will consult a medical or health professional before beginning this or any other weight-loss or physical fitness program.

Rights for publishing this book outside the U.S.A. or in non-English languages are administered by Gospel Light Worldwide, an international not-for-profit ministry. For additional information, please visit www.glww.org, email info@glww.org, or write to Gospel Light Worldwide, 1957 Eastman Avenue, Ventura, CA 93003, U.S.A.

To order copies of this book and other First Place 4 Health products in bulk quantities, please contact us at 1-800-727-5223. You can also order copies from Gospel Light at 1-800-446-7735.

contents

about
the author

Charlotte Davis is the Arkansas First Place 4 Health networking leader and has led groups in Arkansas churches for more than 16 years. She never plans to stop, because God forever changed her life and her priorities when she started her first First Place 4 Health group in 1995. Charlotte is a registered, licensed dietitian and works as the child nutrition director for Searcy Public Schools, a district of approximately 4,000 students. Charlotte and her husband, Tony, have been married for 24 years and have two children, Kayla (19), and Jake (15). Her favorite activities include spending time with her family, serving on the worship team in her church, reading Christian literature, and creating stamped greeting cards to send to her First Place 4 Health friends and family.

about
first place 4 health

*Seek first his kingdom and his righteousness,
and all these things will be given to you as well.*

MATTHEW 6:33

The First Place 4 Health program was developed more than 30 years ago out of a godly desire placed in the hearts of a group of Christians to establish a Christ-centered weight-control program. Since that time, it has evolved into a nationally recognized total-health program.

First Place 4 Health addresses all areas of a person's life—spiritual, mental, emotional and physical—through Bible study, small-group support, accountability, a common sense nutrition plan, exercise, record-keeping and Scripture memory. It is used by people in every U.S. state and many foreign countries. Thousands of lives have been changed!

introduction

We're excited about the booklet that you are holding in your hand for several reasons:

- There is a two-week jump start menu plan to help you kick off your First Place 4 Health journey and aid you during those times when you hit a plateau in your weight-loss efforts.
- There are great tips for healthy eating if you are serious about losing weight and getting healthy.
- There is an alphabetical listing of foods that is based on the U.S. Department of Agriculture's (USDA's) five food groups.

This booklet is not intended to replace the *First Place 4 Health Member's Guide*, but it will be a great resource that you can carry with you to make your First Place 4 Health journey fun and successful.

Blessings,

Carole Lewis,
First Place 4 Health National Director

two-week weight loss jump start plan

Here are 10 things you can do right now to jump start your weight loss journey or when you find yourself at a weight-loss plateau.

1. Pray before you eat anything. Ask God to help you make healthy choices. You can't do it alone, and you don't have to.

2. Weigh yourself. Weigh yourself now—and at the same time each week. Weigh yourself only once per week, as weighing yourself more often can lead to discouragement when you don't see a change quickly.

3. Write down everything you eat. Don't worry about counting it on your Live It Tracker. Just get it down on paper.

4. Don't eat any fried foods. **None. Zero. No excuses.**

5. Eat only low-fat dairy and meat products. **Reduced-fat cheeses are easy to find and taste great. Choose lean cuts of meat and trim any visible fat and skin.**

6. Don't drink any soft drinks, sweetened coffees or juices. **Calorie-heavy soft drinks, coffee drinks and fruit juices can lead to packing on pounds. It's easy to lose track of how many liquid calories you are consuming, so just abstain from all of these during the two-week jump start.**

7. Eat as many vegetables as you want. **You will not gain weight from eating vegetables, so eat as many as you want. (Remember to limit starchy vegetables such as potatoes, corn and peas, as they contain more calories per serving.)**

8. Drink eight ounces of water before every meal and snack. **It will help you feel full faster. Many times, your body will interpret dehydration as hunger.**

9. Get at least eight hours of sleep per night. **Studies have shown that sleep deprivation promotes weight gain.**

10. Exercise at least 30 minutes each day, five times each week. If you can only walk a mile, then only walk a mile. Get serious about it.

These simple steps will kick-start your weight loss efforts. Do each of these for 14 days and you will be back on track. (You can do anything for 14 days!) If you are just beginning your journey with First Place 4 Health, this is a great way to start as you familiarize yourself with all aspects of the program.

two-week weight loss jump start menus

The following pages (14-27) include two weeks of easy menus that you can use to "jump start" your weight loss plan, keep on track, or get back on track whenever you run into a "weight loss plateau"—a time when no matter what you try, you just can't seem to shed any more pounds. Each day's menu is based on approximately 1300–1400 calories and incorporates items from each of the five food groups as recommended by the USDA.

DAY ONE MENU

Breakfast	Snack
1 cup bran flakes cereal 1 cup fat-free milk ½ large banana	1½ oz. 2% cheddar cheese 1 oz. pretzels

Lunch	Snack
Turkey Sandwich* ½ cup baby carrots 2 tbsp. light Ranch dressing	8 oz. sugar-free/fat-free yogurt (any flavor) 1 small apple

Dinner
2 oz. baked or grilled chicken 1 medium (8 oz.) baked potato 1 tbsp. margarine 2 tbsp. fat-free sour cream ½ cup cooked green beans 1 small (1 oz.) whole-wheat dinner roll

* see recipe section on pages 28-32

DAY TWO MENU

Breakfast	Snack
2 regular slices wheat toast 1 tbsp. margarine 2 tbsp. low-sugar jam or jelly 1 medium orange 8 oz. sugar-free/fat-free yogurt	1 oz. string (mozzarella) cheese

Lunch	Snack
*Ham & Cheese Roll-ups** (2) 1 tbsp. light Ranch dressing ½ cup chopped tomato 1 cup shredded lettuce ½ cup grapes	3 cups light popcorn ¼ cup raisins

Dinner
2 oz. ground beef patty (90% lean) ½ cup steamed/boiled broccoli spears or florets ½ cup steamed/boiled yellow squash ½ cup sugar-free pudding

* see recipe section on pages 28-32

DAY THREE MENU

Breakfast	Snack
*Breakfast Sandwich** ½ cup apple juice	½ large banana

Lunch	Snack
*Turkey Sandwich** 1 cup baby carrots 2 tbsp. light Ranch dressing 1 oz. Baked Lay's Potato Chips® (plain)	8 oz. sugar-free/fat-free yogurt

Dinner
1 cup canned turkey chili with beans 1 oz. baked tortilla chips ½ oz. 2% cheddar cheese, shredded 2 cups tossed salad (1½ cups lettuce and ½ cup tomatoes or other vegetables) 1 tbsp. Italian dressing 1 tangerine

* see recipe section on pages 28-32

DAY FOUR MENU

Breakfast	Snack
1 egg (pan-fried/scrambled) 1 regular slice whole-wheat toast 1 tsp. margarine 1 tbsp. low-sugar jam or jelly 8 oz. sugar-free/fat-free yogurt	1 large apple

Lunch	Snack
Stuffed Potato* 15 grapes	1 oz. Wheat Thins® crackers 2 slices (1½ oz. total) 2% American cheese

Dinner
Argentine Corn Chicken* $^1/_3$ cup brown rice 1 cup steamed vegetables

* see recipe section on pages 28-32

DAY FIVE MENU

Breakfast	Snack
1 cup Rice Chex® cereal ½ large banana 1 cup fat-free milk	1 oz. pretzels ½ cup grapes

Lunch	Snack
Fruit & Nut Turkey Salad* ¼ cup light Ranch dressing 6 reduced-fat Ritz crackers	½ large banana 4 graham cracker squares

Dinner
2 oz. grilled or baked salmon fillet ½ cup mashed sweet potato ½ cup boiled/steamed cauliflower florets 1 small (1 oz.) whole-wheat dinner roll 1 tbsp. margarine

* see recipe section on pages 28-32

DAY SIX MENU

Breakfast	Snack
1 (2 ½ oz.) whole-wheat bagel 2 tbsp. light cream cheese 2 tbsp. low-sugar jam or jelly 1 cup fat-free milk ½ grapefruit	8 oz. sugar-free/fat-free yogurt

Lunch	Snack
"Fast food" Grilled Chicken Sandwich (3 oz. chicken, 1½ oz. bun, no mayonnaise or cheese) "Side salad" (1½ cups) fat-free salad dressing (1 oz. packet)	1 cup cantaloupe cubes

Dinner
1 oz. lean smoked ham ½ cup corn ½ cup green beans ½ cup grapes 1 small (1 oz.) whole-wheat dinner roll 1 tsp. margarine ½ cup sugar-free pudding

* see recipe section on pages 28-32

DAY SEVEN MENU

Breakfast	Snack
1 cup Rice Krispies® cereal 1 cup fat-free milk ½ cup orange juice ½ large banana	1 oz. pretzels

Lunch	Snack
2 oz. grilled/baked chicken ½ cup brown rice ½ cup fresh broccoli florets ½ cup fresh cauliflower florets 2 tbsp. light Ranch dressing	½ cup sugar-free pudding

Dinner
Taco Salad ½ cup fruit cocktail

* see recipe section on pages 28-32

DAY EIGHT MENU

Breakfast	Snack
1 egg (scrambled or pan-fried) 1 whole English muffin, toasted 1 tbsp. margarine 1 tbsp. low-sugar jam or jelly 1 cup fat-free milk	½ cup diced peaches ½ cup sugar-free/fat-free yogurt

Lunch	Snack
*Roast Beef Sandwich** ½ cup baby carrots	1 medium fresh pear

Dinner
2 oz. baked/broiled tilapia 1 medium baked potato 1 tbsp. margarine 2 tbsp. fat-free sour cream ½ cup green beans 1 small (1 oz.) whole-wheat dinner roll ½ cup unsweetened applesauce

* see recipe section on pages 28-32

DAY NINE MENU

Breakfast	Snack
1 cup Corn Chex® or Wheat Chex® cereal 1 cup fat-free milk ½ cup strawberries	½ cup apple slices 1 tbsp. peanut butter

Lunch	Snack
1 cup chicken noodle soup 6 Triscuit® crackers 1 slice (¾ oz.) 2% American cheese 1½ cup tossed salad 2 tbsp. fat-free dressing ½ cup fruit cocktail	3 cups light popcorn ½ cup dried cranberries

Dinner
3 oz. grilled or baked chicken breast ½ cup brown rice 1 cup boiled or steamed asparagus ½ cup sugar-free pudding

* see recipe section on pages 28-32

DAY TEN MENU

Breakfast	Snack
1 (4-inch) whole-grain waffle 1 tsp. margarine ¼ cup sugar-free syrup 2 slices turkey bacon 1 medium orange	4 graham cracker squares 6 oz. sugar-free/fat-free yogurt

Lunch	Snack
1 cup canned vegetable soup 6 saltine crackers 1 oz. string (mozzarella) cheese 1½ cups tossed salad 2 tbsp. fat-free dressing 1 small apple	1 cup Cheerios® 1 cup fat-free milk

Dinner
3 oz. baked lean ham ½ cup mashed sweet potato 1 tsp. margarine ½ cup green beans 1 small (1 oz.) whole-wheat dinner roll

* see recipe section on pages 28-32

DAY ELEVEN MENU

Breakfast	Snack
½ cup plain oatmeal ¼ cup fat-free milk ½ cup blueberries 1 slice whole-wheat toast 1 tsp. margarine	3 cups light popcorn ¼ cup raisins

Lunch	Snack
*Chef Salad** ¼ cup light Ranch dressing 1 oz. Wheat Thins® crackers	8 oz. sugar-free/fat-free yogurt

Dinner
3 oz. baked or smoked turkey ½ cup rice (white or brown, cook in chicken broth/boullion   instead of plain water for more flavor) ½ cup cooked spinach ½ cup grapes

* see recipe section on pages 28-32

DAY TWELVE MENU

Breakfast	Snack
1 egg (scrambled or pan-fried) 1 slice whole-wheat toast 1 tsp. margarine 1 tbsp. low-sugar jam or jelly 8 oz. sugar-free/fat-free yogurt	1 medium peach

Lunch	Snack
Turkey Sandwich* 1 cup baby carrots 2 tbsp. light Ranch dressing	2 medium plums

Dinner
1 cup spaghetti noodles ½ cup prepared spaghetti sauce with 2 oz. (½ cup) cooked ground beef (90% lean) (**Note:** spaghetti sauce should have tomatoes listed as the first ingredient) 2 tbsp. Parmesan cheese 1 ½ cups tossed salad 1 tbsp. Italian dressing ½ cup whole kernel corn ½ cup apple slices

* see recipe section on pages 28-32

DAY THIRTEEN MENU

Breakfast	Snack
1 cup Rice Chex® cereal 1 cup fat-free milk ½ large banana	½ cup apple slices 1 slice (¾ oz.) 2% American cheese

Lunch	Snack
PB & J Sandwich* ½ cup baby carrots ½ cup celery sticks 2 tbsp. light Ranch dressing	½ cup sugar-free pudding

Dinner
Chicken Stir-fry* 1 cup rice (white or brown) ½ cup pineapple

* see recipe section on pages 28-32

DAY FOURTEEN MENU

Breakfast	Snack
1 cup shredded wheat cereal 1 cup fat-free milk ½ large banana	½ cup apple slices 1 tbsp. peanut butter

Lunch	Snack

1 cup light/reduced sodium
  beef vegetable soup
6 Triscuit® crackers
1 cup salad (primarily
  Romaine lettuce)
1 tbsp. Italian dressing
½ cup strawberries
	4 graham cracker squares
	½ cup sugar-free pudding

Dinner

2½ oz. grilled sirloin steak (visible fat removed)
1 medium (8 oz.) baked potato
1 tbsp. margarine
2 tbsp. fat-free sour cream
½ cup steamed/boiled asparagus
1 small (1 oz.) whole-wheat dinner roll

* see recipe section on pages 28-32

RECIPES

Turkey Sandwich

2 slices whole-wheat bread
2 oz. deli-sliced turkey
¼ cup lettuce/tomato
1 slice 2% American cheese
1 tbsp. light Miracle Whip®
2 tsp. mustard

Place ingredients between 2 regular-sized slices of bread and serve.

Ham & Cheese Roll-ups

2 (6-inch) whole-wheat tortillas
2 oz. deli-sliced ham
2 slices (1½ oz. total) 2% American cheese

Roll ingredients inside 2 whole-wheat tortillas and serve.

Breakfast Sandwich

1 whole English muffin
1 egg (scrambled or pan-fried with nonstick cooking spray)
1 slice 2% American cheese
½ oz. Canadian bacon

Scramble or pan-fry the egg with nonstick cooking spray. Top with cheese and Canadian bacon. Place between 2 halves of the English muffin and serve.

RECIPES

Stuffed Potato

1 (6-oz.) baked potato
¼ tomato
1 tsp. margarine
¼ cup cooked broccoli florets
1 tbsp. fat-free sour cream
1 oz. turkey bacon (cooked and crumbled)
1 oz. 2% cheddar cheese (shredded)

Bake a potato in the oven at 350° F for 30 to 45 minutes (times will vary based on the size of the potato). Cook and crumble the turkey bacon and shred the cheddar cheese. Scoop out the inside of the baked potato and add tomato, margarine, broccoli florets, sour cream, turkey bacon and cheddar cheese. Mix well and fill potato shell with mixture. Microwave until hot.

Argentine Corn Chicken

4 oz. boneless chicken breast
salt and pepper
1 tsp. vegetable oil
1 onion
1 garlic clove, minced
1 medium tomato (diced)
1 bay leaf
$1/8$ tsp. marjoram
¼ cup corn
4 whole cherry tomatoes

RECITES

RECIPES

Argentine Corn Chicken (con't)

Season the chicken lightly with salt and pepper. Heat the oil in a small skillet. Add boneless chicken breast and cook until tender. Remove from skillet. Sauté onion and garlic clove. Add tomato, bay leaf and marjoram and simmer for 10 minutes. Add corn, cherry tomatoes and chicken. Heat well.

Fruit & Nut Turkey Salad

2 cups mixed leafy salad greens
¼ cup cherry tomatoes
½ oz. walnuts (7 halves)
1 oz. smoked turkey
¼ cup dried cranberries

Chop the walnut halves and dice the smoked turkey. Mix ingredients together and serve.

Taco Salad

2 oz. (½ cup) ground beef (90% lean)
taco seasoning
½ cup black beans
1 cup shredded lettuce
2 oz. baked tortilla chips
1 oz. 2% cheddar cheese
¼ cup chopped tomatoes or chunky salsa
2 tbsp. fat-free sour cream

RECIPES

Taco Salad (con't)

Shred the cheddar cheese. Cook lean ground beef in a pan and drain excess fat. Add taco seasoning and black beans. Combine lettuce, tortilla chips, cheddar cheese with ground beef mixture in a bowl. Top with tomatoes or chunky salsa and sour cream.

Roast Beef Sandwich

2 slices whole-wheat bread
1 oz. deli-style lean roast beef
1 oz. 2% Swiss cheese
lettuce/tomato/pickles (if desired)
2 tsp. spicy mustard

Place ingredients between 2 regular-sized slices of bread and serve.

Chef Salad

2 cups mixed leafy salad greens
1 egg
1 oz. 2% cheddar cheese
¼ cup fresh carrots
¼ cup cherry tomatoes

Boil egg and dice. Shred the cheddar cheese and slice or shred the carrots. Add egg, cheese, carrots and cherry tomatoes to the leafy salad greens and serve.

RECIPES

PB & J Sandwich

2 regular slices whole-wheat bread
2 tbsp. peanut butter
1 tbsp. low-sugar jam or jelly

Place ingredients between 2 regular-sized slices of bread and serve.

Chicken Stir-fry

2 oz. cooked chicken
1 tsp. vegetable oil
1 tbsp. soy sauce
1 cup frozen mixed stir-fry vegetables

Cook the chicken and slice thinly. Stir-fry with vegetable oil and soy sauce until done, and then add frozen mixed stir-fry vegetables. Cook until crisp-tender. Serve with rice (white or brown).

GROCERY LIST

Produce

- ☐ apples
- ☐ asparagus
- ☐ bananas
- ☐ blueberries
- ☐ broccoli
- ☐ cantaloupe
- ☐ carrots
- ☐ carrots, baby
- ☐ cauliflower
- ☐ celery
- ☐ cherry tomatoes
- ☐ corn
- ☐ cranberries
- ☐ garlic cloves
- ☐ grapefruit
- ☐ grapes
- ☐ green beans
- ☐ lettuce (Romaine)
- ☐ onions
- ☐ oranges
- ☐ peaches
- ☐ pears
- ☐ pineapple
- ☐ plums
- ☐ potatoes
- ☐ raisins
- ☐ spinach
- ☐ strawberries
- ☐ sweet potato
- ☐ tangerines
- ☐ tomatoes
- ☐ yellow squash

Baking/Cooking Products

- ☐ nonstick cooking spray
- ☐ vegetable oil

Spices

- ☐ bay leaf
- ☐ marjoram
- ☐ pepper
- ☐ salt

GROCERY LIST

Nuts/Seeds

☐ walnuts

Condiments, Spreads and Sauces

☐ dressing, fat-free   ☐ peanut butter
☐ Italian dressing   ☐ Ranch dressing, light
☐ jam or jelly, low-sugar   ☐ salsa
☐ margarine   ☐ soy sauce
☐ Miracle Whip®, light   ☐ spaghetti sauce*
☐ mustard   ☐ sugar-free syrup
☐ mustard, spicy   ☐ taco seasoning

* first ingredient tomatoes

Breads, Cereals and Pasta

☐ bagel, whole-wheat   ☐ oatmeal, plain
☐ bran flakes   ☐ Rice Chex® cereal
☐ bread, whole-wheat   ☐ Rice Krispies® cereal
☐ brown rice   ☐ shredded wheat cereal
☐ Cheerios®   ☐ spaghetti noodles
☐ Corn Chex®/ Wheat   ☐ tortillas, whole-wheat
   Chex® cereal   ☐ waffles, whole-grain
☐ dinner rolls, whole-wheat   ☐ white rice
☐ English muffins

GROCERY LIST

Canned Foods

- ☐ applesauce, unsweetened
- ☐ beef vegetable soup, reduced sodium
- ☐ black beans
- ☐ chicken broth
- ☐ chicken noodle soup
- ☐ fruit cocktail
- ☐ pickles
- ☐ turkey chili with beans
- ☐ vegetable soup

Dairy Products

- ☐ American cheese (2%)
- ☐ cheddar cheese (2%)
- ☐ cream cheese, light
- ☐ milk, fat-free
- ☐ Parmesan cheese
- ☐ sour cream, fat-free
- ☐ string (mozzarella) cheese
- ☐ sugar-free pudding
- ☐ sugar-free/fat-free yogurt
- ☐ Swiss cheese (2%)

Juices

- ☐ apple juice
- ☐ orange juice

Frozen Foods

- ☐ stir-fry vegetables

GROCERY LIST

Meat and Poultry

- ☐ Canadian bacon
- ☐ chicken
- ☐ eggs
- ☐ ground beef (90% lean)
- ☐ ham, deli-sliced
- ☐ ham, lean
- ☐ roast beef, deli-style, lean
- ☐ salmon
- ☐ sirloin steak
- ☐ tilapia
- ☐ turkey
- ☐ turkey bacon
- ☐ turkey, deli-sliced

Other

- ☐ Baked Lay's Potato Chips®
- ☐ graham crackers
- ☐ popcorn, light
- ☐ Ritz® crackers, reduced-fat
- ☐ pretzels
- ☐ saltine crackers
- ☐ tortilla chips, baked
- ☐ Triscuit® crackers
- ☐ Wheat Thins® crackers

menu tips and guidelines

calorie range

- 1300-1400—This is a good calorie range for beginning first-time members.
- 1500 to 1600—Add 1 ounce meat, ½ cup vegetable and up to 1 ounce more of grains per day. You may also add an additional teaspoon of healthy oils.
- Higher calorie ranges—Refer to the chart in the *First Place 4 Health Member's Guide* (see page 123) or the chart on your Live It Tracker to determine the amount of extra foods to add from each food group.

plan for each day

- Three meals and two snacks may be placed at your discretion. For example, you may want a bedtime snack rather than afternoon snack.

- Add snacks to mealtimes if you do not have the opportunity to eat between meals.

portion sizes

- Portion sizes are very specific. Stick to the recommended serving sizes to insure that you stay within your calorie limit.
- Buy a food scale and a set of measuring cups or spoons to help you learn what each serving size actually looks like.
- Eat everything listed on the menu plans—don't cheat yourself out of nutrients and calories that your body needs.

weights & measurements

- All measurements listed are for the ready-to-eat state of each food. for instance, the oatmeal measurements on pages 64-65 are for after cooking, as are all of the meat measurements.
- It is assumed that you will not add any fat when preparing the items (for instance, no margarine or oil is added to vegetables).

calories

- The jump start menus were planned using foods that are listed in the food list section of this book. Refer to this list when choosing foods so you will know approximately what has been allowed in the meal plan.

- If you don't like (or can't get) a particular food that is listed, just go to the calorie column and choose one from the same group with similar calories.
- Be adventurous . . . give some of the things you've never tried a chance. Long-term success with a healthy lifestyle is often associated with eating a wide variety of foods (this helps to prevent boredom).

substitutions

- When making substitutions, refer to the "tips for healthy eating" section in this book to assure optimal weight loss and nutrition results.
- There are several non-whole grain items listed in the food table, but you can replace any refined/white bread products with whole-grain versions (this is actually encouraged!).

exercise

- Proper diet is only half of the weight loss equation. For complete success, you need to burn off calories through activity and exercise. See pages 180-210 in the *First Place 4 Health Member's Guide* for more information on excercise and strength training.

tips for
healthy eating

The USDA food guide provides suggested amounts of food to consume from the five basic food groups (and from oils) to achieve adequate nutrition at several calorie ranges. The following pages contain tips and nutrition notes so that you can plan what types of foods to eat and what types to avoid for each of the food groups. (For detailed information on each of the food groups, refer to the pages indicated in the *First Place 4 Health Member's Guide*.)

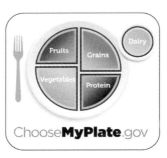

FRUITS
(See pages 126-128 in the *First Place 4 Health Member's Guide*)

Approximate calories (average) for ½ cup of fruit:	40
Choose often:	Fresh and frozen fruits, canned fruits packed in water or juice.
Choose occasionally:	Dried fruits, fruits canned in light syrup, 100% fruit juice, olives, avocados.
What does "occasionally" mean?	Up to ½ cup per *day* of these foods.
Choose seldom:	Fruits canned in heavy syrup, fruits prepared in butter or cream sauce, coconut.
What does "seldom" mean?	No more than ½ cup per *week* of these foods.
Calorie control notes:	If you purchase canned fruits with heavy syrup or light syrup, drain off the syrup and rinse before eating. This will eliminate *most* of the unwanted empty calories.
Nutrition notes:	Strive to include at least one fresh fruit per day, and vary your fruit choices to include lots of colors/textures for optimal nutrition!

VEGETABLES
(See pages 129-132 in the *First Place 4 Health Member's Guide*)

Approximate calories (average) for ½ cup of vegetables:	Non-starchy: 20 Starchy: 80
Choose often:	Fresh or frozen vegetables without added fat (butter or gravy).
Choose occasionally:	Canned vegetables without salt.
What does "occasionally" mean?	Eating these foods *daily* is fine, but try to eat frozen vegetables (rather than canned) as much as possible for optimal nutrition.
Choose seldom:	Canned vegetables with salt, vegetables prepared in butter or cream sauce, fried vegetables.
What does "seldom" mean?	You can eat salted canned vegetables *daily* (it's best to drain the liquid) without affecting weight-loss results, but use with discretion, especially if you have high blood pressure, fluid retention issues, or other medical concerns. Limit eating vegetables that have been fried or prepared in a butter or cream sauce to a maximum of 1 cup per week.
Calorie control notes:	When consuming vegetables that have been fried or prepared in a cream sauce (listed under "seldom"), eliminate at least one teaspoon of healthy oil from your meal plan per ½ cup of those vegetables eaten. Because there is a *wide* variance

VEGETABLES (CONT'D)
(See pages 129-132 in the *First Place 4 Health Member's Guide*)

Calorie control notes (cont'd):	between the calories in starchy versus non-starchy vegetables, limit your intake of starchy vegetables to an *average* of ½ cup per day (maximum 3½ cups per week) to stay within the daily calorie allowance. Don't panic if you are a starchy-vegetable lover—because this is an average, it will allow you to eat a medium baked potato (1 cup) one day a week as long as you avoid eating starchy vegetables on another day that same week. When you are counting beans as meat instead of vegetables, you do not need to consider them in the 3½-cup weekly maximum— the calories are "covered" in the meat serving.
Nutrition notes:	Do *not* avoid starchy vegetables just because of the calories. A sweet potato is one of the higher-calorie starchy vegetables, but it packs a powerful punch with Vitamin A and fiber as compared to many other vegetables. Current research shows that most people should eat at least 3 cups dark green vegetables and 2 cups orange vegetables per week for optimum nutrition—so go for the color!

GRAINS
(See pages 133-137 in the *First Place 4 Health Member's Guide*)

Approximate calories (average) for 1 ounce of grain:	70
Choose often:	Whole-grain breads, bagels, tortillas, pitas, pasta and cereals; oats, brown rice, bulgur, low-fat whole-grain crackers, low-fat popcorn, pretzels.
Choose occasionally:	White bread and pasta that is not whole grain, baked corn tortillas, taco shells, baked chips, granola, regular crackers, fat-free cakes and cookies, biscuits, fig bars, angel food cake; French toast, waffles or pancakes made with whole grain.
What does "occasionally" mean?	Foods on this list may be consumed up to *half* of your grains for each day.
Choose seldom:	Fried chips, croissants, pastry, pies, doughnuts, sweet rolls, snack crackers with hydrogenated oils (trans fats), sweetened breakfast cereals, refined grain products prepared with cream, butter, sugar or cheese sauce.
What does "seldom" mean?	Limit these high-fat grains to 1 ounce maximum per week, and eliminate 2 to 3 teaspoons of healthy oil from your meal plan whenever they are consumed. If you are wondering about a packaged product that has a nutrition label, you will need to

GRAINS (CONT'D)
(See pages 133-137 in the *First Place 4 Health Member's Guide*)

What does "seldom" mean (cont'd)?	eliminate 1 teaspoon of healthy oil from your meal plan for every 5 grams of fat contained in a one ounce portion.
Calorie control notes:	See above.
Nutrition notes:	Try to make at least *half* of the grains you consume whole grains. The easiest way to determine if something qualifies as a whole grain is to check out the ingredient listing. If a whole grain (such as whole-wheat flour, whole corn or whole oats) is listed *first*, then it can qualify!

MILK PRODUCTS
(See pages 138-141 in the *First Place 4 Health Member's Guide*)

Approximate calories (average) for 1 cup of milk:	90
Choose often:	Skim milk, 1% milk and buttermilk, nonfat and low-fat yogurt, nonfat frozen yogurt; part-skim, low-fat and fat-free cheese; low-fat and fat-free cottage cheese, soy milk, soy cheese.
Choose occasionally:	2% milk, 2% cheese, 4% cottage cheese, light cream cheese, light sour cream, low-fat sherbet, processed cheese spreads, light nondairy whipped cream.
What does "occasionally" mean?	Up to one cup equivalent of these foods *daily*.
Choose seldom:	Whole milk, regular cheese, cream, half-and-half, most nondairy creamers, whipped cream, full-fat nondairy whipped cream, full-fat cream cheese, full-fat sour cream, full-fat ice cream, full-fat yogurt.
What does "seldom" mean?	No more than one cup equivalent of these foods *weekly*. See below for calorie control tip.
Calorie control notes:	To keep your calories in line, you may have to "trade off" the items that are most important to you. For instance, if you can handle fat-free

MILK PRODUCTS (CONT'D)
(See pages 138-141 in the *First Place 4 Health Member's Guide*)

Calorie control notes (cont'd):	(skim) milk and fat-free yogurt but can't **stand** fat-free cheese, go with the 2% cheese and count that as your "occasional" item for that day. Also, whenever you go with the 2% items, you will need to eliminate 1 teaspoon of healthy oil from your meal plan for that day for each cup of milk equivalent. In addition, if you choose a "seldom" food (such as regular ice cream), you will need to eliminate **two** teaspoons of healthy oil from your daily meal plan.
Nutrition notes:	Go with fat-free milk products as much as you can to eliminate the unhealthy saturated fat in your diet!

MEAT & BEANS
(See pages 142-145 in the *First Place 4 Health Member's Guide*)

Approximate calories (average) for 1 ounce of meat/beans:	70
Choose often:	Lean cuts of beef and pork, extra-lean ground beef (i.e., 90% to 95% lean), poultry without skin, dried beans and peas, lentils, tofu, egg whites, egg substitutes; baked, broiled, grilled or steamed fish; tuna canned in water.
Choose occasionally:	Lean ground beef (i.e., 85% to 90% lean), whole eggs cooked without fat, fish sticks (baked), tuna canned in oil, poultry with skin, ham, Canadian bacon, chicken nuggets (baked), turkey hot dogs, nuts, nut butters.
What does "occasionally" mean?	No more than ½ of your daily meat allowance should come from this group. For example, if you eat 4 ounces per day of meat, then only *two* of them should come from this specific group.
Choose seldom:	Prime-grade meats, ribs, duck, goose, dark poultry meat, regular ground beef (i.e., 75% to 85% lean), bacon, sausage, pepperoni, whole eggs cooked with fat, bologna, salami, hot dogs, organ meats; fried fish, chicken or beef.

MEAT & BEANS (CONT'D)
(See pages 142-145 in the *First Place 4 Health Member's Guide*)

What does "seldom" mean?	Limit to a maximum of 4 ounces from this group per **week**. See the calorie tip below.
Calorie control notes:	When using the "seldom" foods (e.g., bacon, regular sausage, regular ground beef), be sure to eliminate 1 teaspoon of healthy oil from your meal plan for every ounce in this category that you eat. When choosing beans for your protein source, *do not* count them toward your vegetable allowance that day, for if you do, you will be cheating yourself on calories and nutrients!
Nutrition notes:	If you are not sure whether certain cuts of beef or pork are "lean" (due to no notations on the package), look for the visible fat content. A white exterior and marbling ("specks") within the the flesh of the meat indicate a higher fat content. Choose non-meat protein sources (such as beans and nuts) frequently, as current research shows that consuming these types of food can lower your chances of obtaining many types of chronic diseases.

HEALTHY OILS (See pages 146-148 in the *First Place 4 Health Member's Guide*)	
Approximate calories (average) for 1 teaspoon of oil:	45
Choose often:	Olive oil, canola oil, peanut oil, fat-free mayonnaise.
Choose occasionally:	Safflower, corn, soybean, sesame and sunflower oils; mayonnaise made with canola oil; light or reduced-fat mayonnaise, lower-fat salad dressings, trans fat-free margarine.
What does "occasionally" mean?	It is **best** to use oils in the "often" group, but these oils are okay to use **daily** as long as you follow the guidelines for the maximum number of teaspoons to consume per day.
Choose seldom:	Butter, lard, beef tallow, bacon fat, regular mayonnaise, full-fat salad dressings, shortening, palm kernel and coconut oils, stick margarine or shortening made with hydrogenated oil and containing trans fats.
What does "seldom" mean?	Limit amount to 3 to 4 teaspoons per week to help control saturated fat intake.
Calorie control notes:	Remember that while you will likely not pour these oils out of a bottle at home into your foods, they will be present when you **purchase** certain

HEALTHY OILS (CONT'D)
(See pages 146-148 in the *First Place 4 Health Member's Guide*)

Calorie control notes (cont'd):	products. For example, if you are buying a cracker, baked chips or other grain snack food that contains fat (see the nutrition facts panel), you will need to count one teaspoon of healthy oil for every 5 grams of fat that you consume.
Nutrition notes:	See above.

food list

The *My Food Plan* booklet includes many of the foods we eat every day. Unlike the listing by food group in the *First Place 4 Health Member's Guide*, the foods listed in this book are arranged in easy-to-find alphabetical order. You will find the calories for each food in addition to the tracker information to help you complete your Live It Tracker. The information compiled in this section was taken from information provided by the United States Department of Agriculture.

FRUITS			
Food	Quantity	Tracker Value	Calories
apple slices, dehydrated	¼ cup	½ cup fruit	86
apple, large	1 (8 oz.)	2 cups fruit	116
apple, medium	1 (5-6 oz.)	1¼ cup fruit	72
apple, small	1 (< 4 oz.)	1 cup fruit	53
applesauce, sweetened	½ cup	½ cup fruit	97
applesauce, unsweetened	½ cup	½ cup fruit	52
apricots, canned (light syrup)	6 halves	½ cup fruit	90
apricots, dried	¼ cup	½ cup fruit	86
apricots, fresh	2 medium	½ cup fruit	34
avocado	½ cup cubes	½ cup fruit	120
banana chips	¼ cup	½ cup fruit	66
banana, large	8-inch (5 oz.)	1 cup fruit	121
banana, medium	7-inch (4 oz.)	¾ cup fruit	105
banana, small	6-inch (3 oz.)	½ cup fruit	72
blackberries	½ cup	½ cup fruit	31
blueberries, dried	¼ cup	½ cup fruit	100
blueberries, fresh	½ cup	½ cup fruit	41
boysenberries	½ cup	½ cup fruit	31
cantaloupe	½ cup cubes	½ cup fruit	30
cherries, dried	¼ cup	½ cup fruit	100

FRUITS (CONT'D)

Food	Quantity	Tracker Value	Calories
cherries, fresh	½ cup	½ cup fruit	37
cranberries, dried	¼ cup	½ cup fruit	104
fruit cocktail, canned in juice	½ cup	½ cup fruit	55
fruit cocktail, canned (light syrup)	½ cup	½ cup fruit	64
grapefruit	½ medium	½ cup fruit	41
grapes, seedless	½ cup	½ cup fruit	55
honeydew melon	½ cup cubes	½ cup fruit	32
juice, apple	½ cup	½ cup fruit	56
juice, grape	½ cup	½ cup fruit	77
juice, grapefruit	½ cup	½ cup fruit	47
juice, orange	½ cup	½ cup fruit	53
juice, pineapple	½ cup	½ cup fruit	70
juice, prune	½ cup	½ cup fruit	90
kiwi	½ cup	½ cup fruit	46
mango	½ cup cubes	½ cup fruit	54
nectarine	½ cup slices	½ cup fruit	30
orange, fresh, small	1 (2-inch)	½ cup fruit	42
orange, fresh, medium	1 (2½-inch)	¾ cup fruit	62
orange, fresh, large	1 (3-inch)	1 cup fruit	86
oranges, canned (Mandarin)	½ cup	½ cup fruit	77

FRUITS (CONT'D)

Food	Quantity	Tracker Value	Calories
papaya	½ cup cubes	½ cup fruit	27
peach, fresh	1 medium	½ cup fruit	38
peaches, canned in juice	½ cup	½ cup fruit	55
pear, fresh	1 medium	1 cup fruit	96
pears, canned in juice	½ cup	½ cup fruit	64
pineapple, canned in juice	½ cup	½ cup fruit	60
pineapple, fresh	½ cup	½ cup fruit	37
plum	1 medium	½ cup fruit	30
pomegranate, raw	½ medium	½ cup fruit	52
prunes	¼ cup	½ cup fruit	102
raisins	¼ cup	½ cup fruit	108
raspberries	½ cup	½ cup fruit	32
sorbet, made with fruit	½ cup	½ cup fruit	82
star fruit (Carambola)	½ cup slices	½ cup fruit	17
strawberries, fresh	½ cup	½ cup fruit	23
strawberries, frozen, unsweetened	½ cup (thawed)	½ cup fruit	39
tangerines/clementines	1 medium	½ cup fruit	37
watermelon	½ cup cubes	½ cup fruit	23

FRUITS: FAVORITES

Food	Quantity	Tracker Value	Calories

VEGETABLES

Food	Quantity	Tracker Value	Calories
asparagus	½ cup	½ cup vegetable	20
artichoke	½ cup	½ cup vegetable	42
bean sprouts	½ cup	½ cup vegetable	29
beans, green	½ cup	½ cup vegetable	14
beans, Italian	½ cup	½ cup vegetable	14
beans, wax	½ cup	½ cup vegetable	14
beets	½ cup	½ cup vegetable	37
broccoli, cooked	½ cup	½ cup vegetable	17
broccoli, fresh	½ cup	½ cup vegetable	12
cabbage, cooked	½ cup	½ cup vegetable	17
cabbage, raw	½ cup	½ cup vegetable	14
carrot juice	½ cup	½ cup vegetable	47

VEGETABLES (CONT'D)

Food	Quantity	Tracker Value	Calories
carrots, cooked	½ cup	½ cup vegetable	27
carrots, fresh	½ cup	½ cup vegetable	25
cauliflower, cooked	½ cup	½ cup vegetable	17
cauliflower, raw	½ cup	½ cup vegetable	13
celery, raw	½ cup	½ cup vegetable	8
cucumbers	½ cup	½ cup vegetable	7
eggplant	½ cup	½ cup vegetable	35
greens, variety, cooked	½ cup	½ cup vegetable	18
mushrooms, cooked	½ cup	½ cup vegetable	22
mushrooms, raw	½ cup	½ cup vegetable	8
okra, boiled/steamed (no breading)	½ cup	½ cup vegetable	18
okra, fried (breaded)	½ cup	½ cup vegetable	87
onions, variety, raw	½ cup	½ cup vegetable	34
onions, white or yellow, cooked	½ cup	½ cup vegetable	46
peas and carrots	½ cup	½ cup vegetable	38
peppers, bell, raw	½ cup	½ cup vegetable	9
pumpkin	½ cup	½ cup vegetable	42
sauerkraut	½ cup	½ cup vegetable	14
salsa	½ cup	½ cup vegetable	35
snow peas	½ cup	½ cup vegetable	34

VEGETABLES (CONT'D)

Food	Quantity	Tracker Value	Calories
spaghetti sauce*	½ cup	½ cup vegetable	51
spinach, cooked	½ cup	½ cup vegetable	30
squash, spaghetti	½ cup	½ cup vegetable	19
squash, yellow/summer	½ cup	½ cup vegetable	18
squash, zucchini	½ cup	½ cup vegetable	18
tomato juice	½ cup	½ cup vegetable	11
tomatoes, cooked	½ cup	½ cup vegetable	22
tomatoes, fresh	½ cup	½ cup vegetable	16
turnips, cooked	½ cup	½ cup vegetable	17
vegetable juice (e.g., V-8®)	½ cup	½ cup vegetable	22
vegetable soup with beef, canned	1 cup (water added)	½ cup vegetable	78

* first ingredient tomatoes

VEGETABLES, RAW/LEAFY

Food	Quantity	Tracker Value	Calories
lettuce, escarole	1 cup	½ cup vegetable	8
lettuce, endive	1 cup	½ cup vegetable	8
lettuce, iceberg	1 cup	½ cup vegetable	6
lettuce, romaine	1 cup	½ cup vegetable	8
spinach	1 cup	½ cup vegetable	7

VEGETABLES, STARCHY

Food	Quantity	Tracker Value	Calories
beans, black	½ cup	½ cup vegetable	114
beans, great northern	½ cup	½ cup vegetable	110
beans, kidney	½ cup	½ cup vegetable	105
beans, lima, green/baby	½ cup	½ cup vegetable	104
beans, navy	½ cup	½ cup vegetable	127
beans, pinto	½ cup	½ cup vegetable	110
beans, refried, fat-free	½ cup	½ cup vegetable	100
beans, refried, regular	½ cup	½ cup vegetable	182
chickpeas	½ cup	½ cup vegetable	148
corn, cream style	½ cup	½ cup vegetable	92
corn, whole kernel	½ cup	½ cup vegetable	88
hominy	½ cup	½ cup vegetable	70
lentils	½ cup	½ cup vegetable	110
olives, black	¼ cup	¼ cup vegetable	39
olives, green	¼ cup	¼ cup vegetable	53
peas, black-eyed	½ cup	½ cup vegetable	79
peas, English/green	½ cup	½ cup vegetable	66
peas, purple hull	½ cup	½ cup vegetable	79
plantain	½ cup	½ cup vegetable	137
pork and beans	½ cup	¼ cup vegetable	124

VEGETABLES, STARCHY (CONT'D)

Food	Quantity	Tracker Value	Calories
potatoes, French fries	1 cup	¼ cup vegetable	194
potatoes, white, baked or boiled	1 med. (8 oz.)	1 cup vegetable	121
potatoes, white, mashed*	½ cup	½ cup vegetable	85
soybeans (edamame)	½ cup	½ cup vegetable	127
squash, acorn	½ cup	½ cup vegetable	40
squash, butternut	½ cup	½ cup vegetable	40
sweet potatoes/yams, mashed	½ cup	½ cup vegetable	80
sweet potato, baked	1 large	1 cup vegetable	162
vegetable soup	1 cup	½ cup vegetable	82

* no margarine

VEGETABLES: FAVORITES

Food	Quantity	Tracker Value	Calories

GRAINS			
Food	Quantity	Tracker Value	Calories
animal crackers	1 oz.	1 oz. grain	127
bagel, cinnamon raisin	1 small	2½ oz. grain	189
bagel, white, plain	1 small	2½ oz. grain	181
bagel, whole-wheat	1 small	2½ oz. grain	173
barley, cooked	½ cup	1 oz. grain	99
biscuit, canned	1 small	½ oz. grain	66
biscuit, canned	1 medium	1 oz. grain	100
bread, French	1 regular slice	1 oz. grain	59
bread, multi-grain	1 regular slice	1 oz. grain	65
bread, rye	1 regular slice	1 oz. grain	67
bread, white, "diet"	1 thin slice	½ oz. grain	48
bread, white, regular	1 regular slice	1 oz. grain	69
bread, whole-wheat, "diet"	1 thin slice	½ oz. grain	54
bread, whole-wheat, regular	1 regular slice	1 oz. grain	69
bulgar (bulghur), cooked	½ cup	1 oz. grain	56
bun, hamburger	1 medium	1½ oz. grain	120
bun, hot dog	1 medium	1½ oz. grain	120
cake, with frosting	1/12 sheet cake	1½ oz. grain	400
cereal, all bran	½ cup	1 oz. grain	78
cereal, bran flakes	1 cup	1 oz. grain	144

GRAINS (CONT'D)

Food	Quantity	Tracker Value	Calories
cereal, Cheerios®	1 cup	1 oz. grain	111
cereal, corn flakes	1 cup	1 oz. grain	90
cereal, Corn/Wheat Chex®	1 cup	1 oz. grain	143
cereal, Grape Nuts®	¼ cup	1 oz. grain	98
cereal, Kashi®, puffed	1 cup	1 oz. grain	88
cereal, puffed wheat	1 cup	½ oz. grain	44
cereal, raisin bran	1 cup	1 oz. grain	195
cereal, Rice Chex®	1 cup	1 oz. grain	124
cereal, Rice Krispies®	1 cup	1 oz. grain	94
cereal, shredded wheat	½ cup	1 oz. grain	85
chips, tortilla, baked	1 cup	1 oz. grain	87
chips, tortilla, regular (fried)	1 cup	1½ oz. grain plus 2 tsp. healthy oil	160
cornbread	1 med. muffin	1½ oz. grain	174
couscous, cooked	½ cup	1 oz. grain	87
crackers, cheese flavored	½ cup	1 oz. grain	133
crackers, cheese flavored, red. fat	½ cup	1 oz. grain	100
crackers, Ritz®	6 rounds	1 oz. grain	90
crackers, Ritz®, reduced fat	6 rounds	1 oz. grain	71
crackers, saltines	6 crackers	1 oz. grain	78

GRAINS (CONT'D)

Food	Quantity	Tracker Value	Calories
crackers, Triscuits®	6 crackers	1 oz. grain	106
crackers, Wheat Thins®	14 crackers	1 oz. grain	133
granola bar	1 bar	1 oz. grain	90
Cream of Wheat®, cooked	½ cup	1 oz. grain	55
croissant	1 medium	2 oz. grain	251
doughnut, cake-type, frosted	1 medium	1 oz. grain	251
doughnut, cake-type, unfrosted	1 medium	1 oz. grain	198
doughnut, raised, frosted	1 medium	1 oz. grain	275
doughnut, raised, jelly-filled	1 medium	1 oz. grain	221
doughnut, raised, unfrosted	1 medium	1 oz. grain	242
English muffin, white	½ medium	1 oz. grain	68
English muffin, whole-wheat	½ medium	1 oz. grain	65
graham crackers	4 squares	1 oz. grain	118
granola bar	1 bar	½ oz. grain	130
granola bar, low-fat	1 bar	½ oz. grain	95
granola, low-fat	½ cup	1 oz. grain	209
granola, regular	½ cup	1 oz. grain	299
grits, hominy, cooked	½ cup	1 oz. grain	56
muffin, blueberry or banana	1 medium	2½ oz. grain	295
oatmeal, flavored, cooked with water	½ cup	1 oz. grain	106

GRAINS (CONT'D)

Food	Quantity	Tracker Value	Calories
oatmeal, plain, cooked with water	½ cup	1 oz. grain	73
pancakes, white	1 (5-inch)	1 oz. grain	91
pancakes, whole-wheat	1 (5-inch)	1 oz. grain	91
pasta, regular (noodles, macaroni)	½ cup cooked	1 oz. grain	98
pasta, whole-wheat	½ cup cooked	1 oz. grain	86
pita	1 (5½-inch)	2 oz. grain	124
popcorn, "light""	3 cups	1 oz. grain	97
popcorn, butter/theater style	3 cups	1 oz. grain	219
pretzels, hard	½ cup	1 oz. grain	76
pretzels, soft	1 medium	4 oz. grain	194
raisin bread	1 reg. slice	1 oz. grain	71
rice, brown, cooked	½ cup	1 oz. grain	107
rice, white, cooked	½ cup	1 oz. grain	102
rice, wild	½ cup	1 oz. grain	65
rice cake	.3 oz.	½ oz. grain	35
roll, white	1 small	1 oz. grain	78
roll, whole-wheat	1 small	1 oz. grain	82
soup, chicken noodle (water added)	1 cup	½ oz. grain	75
taco shells	2 shells	1 oz. grain	124
tortillas, corn	1 (6-inch)	1 oz. grain	53

GRAINS (CONT'D)

Food	Quantity	Tracker Value	Calories
tortillas, white flour	1 (6-inch)	1 oz. grain	110
tortillas, whole-wheat	1 (6-inch)	1 oz. grain	70
waffles, bran/multi-grain/wheat	1 (4-inch)	1 oz. grain	115
waffles, frozen	1 (4-inch)	1 oz. grain	103

GRAINS: FAVORITES

Food	Quantity	Tracker Value	Calories

MILK PRODUCTS

Food	Quantity	Tracker Value	Calories
buttermilk, cultured, fat-free	1 cup	1 cup milk	98
cheese spread, Velveeta®	1 oz.	½ cup milk	80
cheese spread, Velveeta® (2%)	1 oz.	¾ cup milk	60
cheese, American (2%)	1 slice (¾ oz.)	½ cup milk	50
cheese, American, fat-free	1 slice (¾ oz.)	½ cup milk	30
cheese, American, regular	1 slice (¾ oz.)	$1/3$ cup milk	70

MILK PRODUCTS (CONT'D)

Food	Quantity	Tracker Value	Calories
cheese, cheddar (2%)	1 oz.	$2/3$ cup milk	80
cheese, cheddar, fat-free	1 oz.	$2/3$ cup milk	42
cheese, cheddar, regular	1 oz.	$2/3$ cup milk	114
cheese, cottage, low-fat (1%)	½ cup	¼ cup milk	81
cheese, cottage, regular (4%)	½ cup	¼ cup milk	108
cheese, cream, fat-free	2 oz.	¾ cup milk	52
cheese, feta/goat	¼ cup	¾ cup milk	99
cheese, mozzarella, part-skim	1 oz.	$2/3$ cup milk	86
cheese, parmesan, grated	2 tbsp.	½ cup milk	44
cheese, ricotta, regular	¼ cup	½ cup milk	96
cheese, Swiss, regular	1 oz.	$2/3$ cup milk	113
cheese, Swiss (2%)	1 oz.	$2/3$ cup milk	51
hot cocoa mix, made with water	1 packet	¼ cup milk	113
hot cocoa mix, sugar-free, with water	1 packet	¼ cup milk	57
ice cream, light/reduced fat	1 cup	¾ cup milk	216
ice cream, regular	1 cup	¼ cup milk	267
milk, dry (powdered)	$1/3$ cup	1 cup milk	147
milk, evaporated, fat-free/skim	½ cup	1 cup milk	100
milk, evaporated, whole	½ cup	1 cup milk	160
milk, fat-free/skim	1 cup	1 cup milk	83

MILK PRODUCTS (CONT'D)

Food	Quantity	Tracker Value	Calories
milk, low-fat (1%)	1 cup	1 cup milk	102
milk, reduced fat (2%)	1 cup	1 cup milk	122
milk, whole	1 cup	1 cup milk	140
pudding, sugar-free (fat-free milk)	½ cup	½ cup milk	81
pudding, sweetened (fat-free milk)	½ cup	½ cup milk	105
sour cream, fat-free	1 cup	¾ cup milk	168
yogurt, fat-free/sugar free, flavored	1 cup	1 cup milk	98
yogurt, frozen, low-fat	1 cup	¾ cup milk	214
yogurt, frozen, low-fat/sugar-free	1 cup	¾ cup milk	199
yogurt, low-fat, flavored	1 cup	1 cup milk	193
yogurt, plain	1 cup	1 cup milk	138

MILK PRODUCTS: FAVORITES

Food	Quantity	Tracker Value	Calories

MEAT & BEANS

Food	Quantity	Tracker Value	Calories
almonds	½ oz. (12)	1 oz. meat plus 1 tsp. healthy oil	82
anchovies	2 oz.	1½ oz. meat	95
bacon, pork	2 slices	½ oz. meat	87
bacon, turkey	2 slices	1 oz. meat	84
beans, black	¼ cup	1 oz. meat	57
beans, great northern	¼ cup	1 oz. meat	55
beans, kidney	¼ cup	1 oz. meat	53
beans, navy	¼ cup	1 oz. meat	64
beans, pinto	¼ cup	1 oz. meat	55
beans, refried, fat-free	¼ cup	1 oz. meat	50
beans, refried, regular	¼ cup	1 oz. meat	91
beef, lean steak or roast	1 oz.	1 oz. meat	56
beef, ground, 80% lean (chuck)	1 oz.	1 oz. meat	75
beef, ground, 90% lean	1 oz.	1 oz. meat	60
beef, ground, 95% lean	1 oz.	1 oz. meat	50
beef, roast, deli-sliced	1 oz.	1 oz. meat	50
bratwurst	1 oz.	1 oz. meat	113
Canadian bacon	1 oz.	1 oz. meat	43
corn dog	1 corn dog	1½ oz. meat plus 1 oz. grain	280

MEAT & BEANS (CONT'D)

Food	Quantity	Tracker Value	Calories
cashews	½ oz. (9)	1 oz. meat plus 1 tsp. healthy oil	83
chicken, dark meat, no skin	1 oz.	1 oz. meat	66
chicken, fried, with skin	1 oz.	1 oz. meat	80
chicken, white meat, no skin	1 oz.	1 oz. meat	55
chickpeas	¼ cup	1 oz. meat	74
chili, canned (turkey with beans)	1 cup	2-3 oz. meat	210
crab	2 oz. lump	2 oz. meat	40
egg whites	2 whites	1 oz. meat	34
egg, whole, boiled/poached (no fat)	1 whole	1 oz. meat	78
egg, whole, fried	1 whole	1 oz. meat	89
fish, baked (not breaded/battered)	1 oz.	1 oz. meat	41
fish, salmon, baked or broiled	1 oz.	1 oz. meat	48
fish, salmon, smoked	1 oz.	1 oz. meat	33
ham, pork, deli, extra lean	1 oz.	1 oz. meat	37
ham, pork, deli, regular	1 oz.	1 oz. meat	45
ham, pork, smoked	1 oz.	1 oz. meat	45
hazelnuts/filberts	½ oz. (10)	1 oz. meat plus 1 tsp. healthy oil	88
hot dog wiener, low-fat	1 wiener	2 oz. meat	92
hot dog wiener, regular	1 wiener	1½ oz. meat	175

MEAT & BEANS (CONT'D)

Food	Quantity	Tracker Value	Calories
hummus	¼ cup	1½ oz. meat	109
lentils, cooked	¼ cup	1 oz. meat	55
lobster	1 oz.	1 oz. meat	28
energy bar, average	1 bar	1 oz. meat plus 1 oz. grain	180
mixed nuts	½ oz.	1 oz. meat	88
oysters	12 medium	2½ oz. meat	69
peanut butter	1 tbsp.	1 oz. meat plus 1 tsp. healthy oil	96
peanuts	½ oz.	1 oz. meat plus 1 tsp. healthy oil	85
pecans	½ oz. (10 halves)	1 oz. meat plus 2 tsp. healthy oil	98
pistachios	¼ cup (in shell)	1 oz. meat plus 1 tsp. healthy oil	82
pork loin, baked/broiled/grilled	1 oz.	1 oz. meat	59
sausage, polish	¼ cup slices	1 oz. meat	117
sausage, pork, Brown & Serve®	1 patty	½ oz. meat	107
sausage, turkey, link	¼ cup slices	1 oz. meat	59
scallops, baked/broiled/grilled	1 oz.	1 oz. meat	37
seeds, flax	2 tbsp.	1 oz. meat plus 1 tsp. healthy oil	90

MEAT & BEANS (CONT'D)

Food	Quantity	Tracker Value	Calories
seeds, sunflower	½ oz.	1 oz. meat plus 1 tsp. healthy oil	81
shrimp, broiled/grilled/sauteed	1 oz.	1 oz. meat	43
shrimp, fried, battered	2 oz.	1 oz. meat	91
shrimp, steamed/boiled	1 oz.	1 oz. meat	39
soybeans	¼ cup	1 oz. meat	64
spam	2 oz.	2 oz. meat	180
tofu	¼ cup	1 oz. meat	38
tuna, canned in oil	¼ cup	1 oz. meat	56
tuna, canned in water	¼ cup	1 oz. meat	33
turkey or chicken, deli-sliced	1 oz.	1 oz. meat	29
turkey, ground	1 oz.	1 oz. meat	65
turkey, roasted, white meat	1 oz.	1 oz. meat	44
turkey, roasted, white/dark mix	1 oz.	1 oz. meat	47
vegetable beef soup, canned	1 cup (water added)	½ oz. meat	78
veggie burger	1 patty	2 oz. meat	110
veggie dog	1 dog	2 oz. meat plus 1 tsp. healthy oil	163
veggie crumbles	2 oz.	2 oz. meat	110
walnuts	½ oz. (7 halves)	1 oz. meat plus 1 tsp. healthy oil	93

MEAT & BEANS: FAVORITES

Food	Quantity	Tracker Value	Calories

HEALTHY OILS

Food	Quantity	Tracker Value	Calories
margarine, stick, light	1 tbsp.	1 tsp. oil	50
margarine, tub, light	1 tbsp.	1 tsp. oil	50
margarine, tub, regular	1 tsp.	1 tsp. oil	34
mayonnaise, light	1 tbsp.	1 tsp. oil	36
mayonnaise, regular	1 tbsp.	2 tsp. oil	99
oil, vegetable (canola, corn, soybean)	1 tsp.	1 tsp. oil	40
salad dressing, blue cheese	1 tbsp.	2 tsp. oil	98
salad dressing, Italian, regular	1 tbsp.	1 tsp. oil	43
salad dressing, plain (Miracle Whip®)	1 tbsp.	1 tsp. oil	57
salad dressing, plain, light	2 tbsp.	1 tsp. oil	48
salad dressing, Ranch, light	2 tbsp.	1 tsp. oil	48
salad dressing, Ranch, regular	1 tbsp.	2 tsp. oil	71
salad dressing, Thousand Island, regular	1 tbsp.	1 tsp. oil	58

HEALTHY OILS: FAVORITES

Food	Quantity	Tracker Value	Calories

"EXTRAS"
(DO NOT CONTRIBUTE SIGNIFICANT TRACKER VALUE QUANTITIES TO THE FOOD GROUPS LISTED ABOVE)

Food	Quantity	Tracker Value	Calories
barbeque sauce	2 tbsp.	N/A	24
butter	1 tsp.	N/A	36
cocktail sauce	¼ cup	N/A	55
coffee creamer, dry	1 tsp.	N/A	10
coffee creamer, liquid	1 tbsp.	N/A	20
cool whip	2 tbsp.	N/A	41
cream cheese, light	2 tbsp.	N/A	69
cream cheese, regular	2 tbsp.	N/A	101
cream/white sauce	¼ cup	N/A	91
gravy, beef, from mix	¼ cup	N/A	31
gravy, chicken, from mix	¼ cup	N/A	47

"EXTRAS" (CONT'D) (DO NOT CONTRIBUTE SIGNIFICANT TRACKER VALUE QUANTITIES TO THE FOOD GROUPS LISTED ABOVE)			
Food	Quantity	Tracker Value	Calories
gravy, cream/milk	¼ cup	N/A	88
gravy, sausage	¼ cup	N/A	94
half and half	2 tbsp.	N/A	39
honey	1 tbsp.	N/A	64
jelly or jam, low sugar	1 tbsp.	N/A	26
Jell-O®, sugar-free	3½ oz. cup	N/A	4
ketchup	1 tbsp.	N/A	14
margarine, stick, regular (hard)	1 tsp.	N/A	35
mustard	1 tsp.	N/A	3
potato chips, baked	1 cup	N/A	94
potato chips, regular/fried	1 cup	N/A	107
salad dressing, Ranch, fat-free	2 tbsp.	N/A	36
shortening, vegetable	1 tsp.	N/A	37
soup, cream of chicken, reduced fat	½ cup (undiluted)	N/A	70
soup, cream of chicken, reduced fat	1 can (10 oz.)	N/A	175
soup, cream of chicken, regular	½ cup (undiluted)	N/A	117
soup, cream of mushroom, reduced fat	½ cup (undiluted)	N/A	70
soup, cream of mushroom, reduced fat	1 can (10 oz.)	N/A	175
soup, cream of mushroom, regular	½ cup (undiluted)	N/A	131

"EXTRAS" (CONT'D)
(DO NOT CONTRIBUTE SIGNIFICANT TRACKER VALUE QUANTITIES TO THE FOOD GROUPS LISTED ABOVE)

Food	Quantity	Tracker Value	Calories
sour cream, fat-free	2 tbsp.	N/A	20
sour cream, light	2 tbsp.	N/A	44
sour cream, regular	2 tbsp.	N/A	62
sugar, granulated	1 tsp.	N/A	16
sweet and sour sauce	2 tbsp.	N/A	28
syrup, sugar-free	¼ cup	N/A	24
whipped topping, non-dairy, fat-free	2 tbsp.	N/A	15
whipped topping, non-dairy, fat-free	8 oz. tub	N/A	360
whipped topping, non-dairy, light	2 tbsp.	N/A	20
whipped topping, non-dairy, light	8 oz. tub	N/A	480
whipped topping, non-dairy, regular	2 tbsp.	N/A	30
whipped topping, non-dairy, regular	8 oz. tub	N/A	720

"EXTRAS": FAVORITES

Food	Quantity	Tracker Value	Calories
		N/A	
		N/A	
		N/A	
		N/A	
		N/A	
		N/A	

Experience a First Place 4 Health Miracle

Teaching New Members Is Easy!

The First Place 4 Health Kit contains everything members need to live healthy, lose weight, make friends, and experience spiritual growth. With each resource, members will make positive changes in their thoughts and emotions, while transforming the way they fuel and recharge their bodies and relate to God.

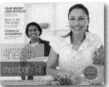

97808307.45890
$99.99 (A $145 Value!)

Member's Kit Contains:
- First Place 4 Health Hardcover Book
- Emotions & Eating DVD
- First Place 4 Health Member's Guide
- First Place 4 Health Prayer Journal
- Simple Ideas for Healthy Living
- First Place 4 Health Tote Bag
- Food on the Go Pocket Guide
- Why Should a Christian Be Physically Fit? DVD

lost 74
pounds in 9
months!

Abby Meloy,
New Life Christian Fellowship
Lake City, Florida

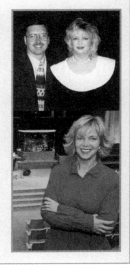

I am thankful for the First Place program. As a pastor's wife who remained at the 200-pound (+) mark for seven years, I can now say I am 135 pounds, a size 8, and I have maintained this weight.

In the beginning, I did not want to try First Place 4 Health. I did not want to weigh my food or take the time to learn the measurements, but the ladies in my church wanted the program, and I was a size 18/20, so I gave it a shot. After our first session, I was 27 pounds lighter and had new insights that my body is the temple of the Holy Spirit. It took me 9 months and 3 sessions to lose 74 pounds.

My new lifestyle has influenced my husband to lose 20 pounds and my 13-year-old daughter to lose 35 pounds. We are able to carry out the work of the ministry with much less fatigue. I now teach others in my church the First Place program and will be forever grateful that the Lord brought it into my life.

Influence Others to Put Christ First in Their Lives

Starting a Group Is Easy!

The First Place 4 Health Group Starter Kit includes everything you need to start and confidently lead your group into healthy living, weight loss, friendships, and spiritual growth. You will find lesson plans, training DVDs, a user-friendly food plan and other easy-to-use tools to help you lead members to a new way of thinking about health and Christ through a renewed mind, emotions, body and spirit.

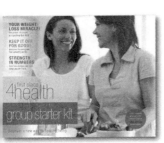

Group Starter Kit Contains:
- A Complete Member's Kit with Member Navigation Sheet
- First Place 4 Health Leader's Guide
- Seek God First Bible Study
- First Place 4 Health Orientation and and Food Plan DVD
- How to Lead with Excellence DVD

978.08307.45906
$199.99 (A $256 value!)

Jim Clayton, D.Min.
Senior Pastor, Dixie Lee Baptist Church
Lenoir City, Tennessee

As a pastor, the changes in my life as a result of First Place 4 Health have provided me the opportunity to more adequately equip our church family to see themselves individually as God's temple. I know of no other health program available with the biblical and doctrinal integrity provided by First Place 4 Health. I lost 80 pounds in 1993 after joining First Place 4 Health and have kept it off for the last sixteen years.

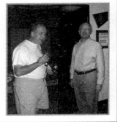